Contents

Prologue ....

What is MRCP? ....

Who should sit MRCP? 6

When should I sit MRCP Part 1? 7

When should I sit MRCP Part 2? 9

Where are the written exams held? 11

How much do the exams cost? 12

Why MRCP? 13

How difficult is MRCP? 15

The difference between attempting and passing 19

Resources: practice makes perfect 21

The main difference between Part I & Part II written 25

Thought process 26

Mixed Category Revision 27

Time allocation 28

High yield facts & pattern recognition 31

Variety 33

Logistics 36

Day of your exam 37

Failing - What Next? 39

Prologue

Although there are various comprehensive books reinforcing the medical knowledge required to pass the MRCP written exams, there is surprisingly little information describing the **overall strategy** one should adopt.

A good analogy is that of a soldier: despite the fact he may win some battles by becoming a proficient fighter and user of weapons, he cannot realistically expect to continue doing so unless he familiarises himself with the surrounding **terrain** upon which the war is being fought. Likewise, to attain the MRCP diploma, you'll be required to demonstrate hard work and reinforce the medical knowledge you accrued throughout medical school and clinical practice. In addition you must ensure that you familiarise yourself with the "terrain" of this exam.

The purpose of this guide is to act as that **compass**. It serves to take you through the terrain of the MRCP written exams where hopefully your hard work will shine through.

This **2020 edition** takes into account the **new MRCP Part 2 Written format** but the original writings still hold true to this day.

What is MRCP?

MRCP stands for the **Membership of the Royal College of Physicians**. Once a candidate passes all three parts (Parts I and II written, and PACES) of their exam then they're elected to membership and awarded the **MRCP diploma**.

Part I consists of **two 3-hour papers** separated by a 1 hour break. Each paper comprises approximately 100 questions, **totalling 200 questions in 6 hours**. Each question generally contains a stem followed by five options, from which you have to pick the best one. Thus it is called **best-of-five (BOF)**. A typical question example is as follows:

You are the cardiology CT1. An 82-year-old lady attends clinic with longstanding confirmed hypertension. Blood pressure today is 182/95. Her medication history includes amlodipine 10mg OD. Assuming she is fully compliant with her medication and this is a true reading what advice would you give her?

- A. Add doxazosin
- B. Add ramipril
- C. Ignore reading and reassure
- D. Add bendroflumethiazide
- E. Add bisoprolol

Each year MRCPUK dedicates a specific number of questions to each specialty to ensure coverage of all specialties. From 2020 this is divided as follows:

Specialty	Marks	% of exam
Cardiology	14	7
Clinical Pharmacology & Therapeutics	15	7.5
Clinical Sciences	25	12.5
Dermatology	8	4
Endocrinology, Diabetes & Metabolic Medicine	14	7
Gastroenterology & Hepatology	14	7
Geriatric Medicine	8	4
Haematology	10	5
Infectious Diseases	14	7
Neurology	14	7
Oncology	5	2.5
Medical Ophthalmology	4	2
Palliative Medicine & End of Life Care	4	2
Psychiatry	9	4.5
Renal Medicine	14	7
Respiratory Medicine	14	7
Rheumatology	14	7
	200	**100**

MRCP Part 1 format

The clinical sciences section is further subdivided as follows:

	Marks	% of exam
Cell, Molecular & Membrane Biology	2	1
Clinical Anatomy	3	1.5
Clinical Biochemistry & Metabolism	4	2
Clinical Physiology	4	2
Genetics	3	1.5
Immunology	4	2
Statistics, Epidemiology & Evidence-based Medicine	5	2.5
	25	**12.5**

MRCP Part 1, Clinical Sciences breakdown

Part II written has a similar format and used to consist of three 3-hour papers when I sat it. This resulted in a mammoth exam totalling 270 marks over 9 hours which was done over the course of 2 days!

You'll be glad to hear that they scrapped this idea and now you're only expected to sit **two 100-mark papers over the course of 1 day**, similar to its part 1 counterpart. Part II continues the theme of focusing on the "major" medical specialties:

Specialty	Marks	% of exam
Cardiology	19	9.5
Dermatology	9	4.5
Endocrinology & Metabolic Medicine	19	9.5
Gastroenterology	19	9.5
Geriatric Medicine	9	4.5
Haematology	9	4.5
Infectious Diseases & GUM	19	9.5
Neurology	17	8.5
Nephrology	19	9.5
Oncology & Palliative Medicine	9	4.5
Ophthalmology	3	1.5
Psychiatry	3	1.5
Respiratory Medicine	19	9.5
Rheumatology	9	4.5
Therapeutics & Toxicology	18	9
	200	**100**

MRCP Part 2 format

The specific breakdown of both exams is very important to our strategy and we will discuss this shortly.

Who should sit MRCP?

Contrary to popular belief, candidates who attempt MRCP do not necessarily have to be aspiring physicians. In fact I have come across aspiring general practitioners; anaesthetists, radiologists and even a fully qualified pathologist who decided to retrain in general medicine!

However, the vast majority of candidates reading this guide will be **aspiring physicians**.

When should I sit MRCP Part 1?

As soon as aspiring physicians overcome the hurdle of transitioning from medical student to doctor, one of the first questions they ask themselves is "When should I sit MRCP?".

Fortunately this difficult question has been made slightly easier by MRCPUK: "Part 1 is the **entry-level examination** accessible to doctors with a **minimum of 12-months' postgraduate experience** in **medical employment**."

This essentially means that the earliest you can attempt Part 1 is at the **beginning** (generally September) **of foundation year 2 (FY2).** Some deaneries and royal colleges go one step further and advise you to accrue more medical experience and wait until **internal medicine training (IMT)***, prior to attempting Part 1. This is evidenced at IMT applications where you'll find no additional shortlisting points awarded for an attempt or even a pass at the exam.

With hindsight I felt my foundation years were the least demanding in terms of **mental** and **emotional workload** and **eportfolio requirements**. Attempting MRCP Part 1 in early-mid FY2 isn't a bad idea at all. Just be wary that if you choose this route, you'll find yourself also juggling IMT applications. Multitasking never ends well for me...

A common concern with sitting Part 1 in FY2 is **perceived lack of experience** but personally, I never felt significant "shop floor time" was required for this initial hurdle. The exam can be considered as purely theoretical meaning a combination of familiarity with guidelines and repeating a relatively large number of practice questions should suffice.

If you're reading this having bested Part 1, take a breather and congratulate yourself first...but not too much. You're probably not going to like what follows.

*Previously IMT was called core medical training

When should I sit MRCP Part 2?

One of the biggest regrets I hear from Part 2 candidates is taking a break after passing Part 1. On the flipside ask five registrars on their opinion and you'll probably receive five different answers. There's a time and place to take breaks – in fact I'm all for taking your time and *enjoying the process*.

The major problem I have nowadays is never living in the present and *always striving for the next thing*. After attaining the MRCP diploma and getting a ST3 training post in respiratory I recall there was a major lull where I just went to work, enjoyed time outside work, rinse and repeat. I felt like I was wasting a lot of time but in reality, there is always a next thing - the respiratory consultant exam which I also passed. Just remember there will always be a next thing and you should **relax**, **enjoy yourself** and most importantly **congratulate yourself** when things do go well.

The only caveat to this rule is that I would strongly recommend an attempt at Part 2 written immediately after passing Part 1. I wouldn't particularly worry about under-preparation because realise that the pass mark for Part 2 written is significantly lower than Part 1 and...you'll be fine.

All the work you did for Part 1 is half the battle.

Another reason for passing Part 1 and 2 quickly and consecutively is that this will allow you plenty of time to improve your clinical skills prior to tackling MRCP PACES. It will also give you the opportunity for second attempts and less pressure when ST3/4 applications rear their ugly head.

As a side note, IMT applications have only recently been phased in. Depending on which specialty (ST3/4) you wish to apply for IMT will have a duration of 2 or 3 years. Accordingly, you'll also be given 2 or 3 years to attain your MRCP diploma.

For example, if you wish to become an endocrinologist, IMT will be 3 years for you and therefore you'll have 3 years to attain MRCP. On the other hand, if you wish to do haematology then IMT will take 2 years and you'll only have 2 years to attain MRCP. For the 3 year IMT specialties although you're expected to pass MRCP (UK) by end of year 2, you can still progress to year 3 if you achieve all the other necessary clinical competencies.

If you follow this guideline and work diligently then you may find yourself in the enviable position of having passed both written exams by the start of CT1.

However, if you're like me and wish someone gave you all this advice when you were a foundation trainee then do not despair. I passed all three MRCP exams within 10 months during CT1 so it's very achievable if you're willing to sacrifice some things.

Where are the written exams held?

The UK exams are distributed country-wide and venues have included science centres, churches, universities, hospitals and even rugby/football stadiums!

How much do the exams cost?

In 2020 UK charges £419 for each written exam.

The international centres charge £594 for each written exam.

PACES costs £657 in the UK.

The international PACES centres vary their fees and will be in their local currency. Check the MRCPUK website for more info.

Why MRCP?

Good question. Why should I pay £1,495 to sit these three exams? This figure does not include training websites, courses and resits!

For non-physicians, attempting MRCP Part I demonstrates your holistic approach as a doctor.

As a result of being attracted to medicine, my medical knowledge is strong but often I find everything else is a relative knowledge gap. If you have time and you wish to become a better doctor, it's worth studying for MRCP. You may not retain all the revision if you go on and pursue a different specialty but some **key concepts** will stick with you forever.

In particular, general practitioners may have had as little as 4 months of general medicine during FY1 followed by 6 months during GP training before being expected to recognise complex pathology on a daily basis. 10 months is hardly enough time to become adept at one medical specialty, let alone all of them!

For aspiring physicians, passing all three parts of MRCP is not an option. If you wish to progress to **higher specialist training** in any of the below medical specialties, then attaining the MRCP diploma is one of the key requirements:

Acute Internal Medicine

Allergy
Audiovestibular Medicine
Aviation and Space Medicine
Cardiology
Clinical Genetics
Clinical Neurophysiology
Clinical Pharmacology & Therapeutics
Combined Infection Training
Dermatology
Endocrinology & Diabetes Mellitus
Gastroenterology
General Internal Medicine
Genitourinary Medicine
Geriatric Medicine
Haematology
Immunology
Infectious Diseases & Tropical Medicine
Medical Microbiology
Medical Oncology
Medical Ophthalmology
Metabolic Medicine
Neurology
Nuclear Medicine
Palliative Medicine
Pharmaceutical Medicine
Rehabilitation Medicine
Renal Medicine
Respiratory Medicine
Rheumatology
Sport & Exercise Medicine
Stroke Medicine

How difficult is MRCP?

Just how difficult is MRCP? The answer to this question depends on who you ask!

In the old MRCP days of negative marking, when candidates answered a question incorrectly, they would've lost marks (as opposed to simply being awarded a zero nowadays).

Thankfully, **negative marking no longer exists** in MRCP but as you can see, with the exception of maybe Part 2, the pass rates remain very low:

		UK trainees	"Other" trainees
MRCP Part 1	2014	48.5%	37.1%
	2015	60.9%	48.3%
	2016	59.7%	41.9%
	2018	51.2%	39.5%
	2019	**57.8%**	**40.2%***
MRCP Part 2	2015	82.2%	73%
	2016	80.6%	69.5%
	2018	64.9%	57.7%
	2019	**73.8%**	**59.9%***
MRCP PACES	2015	61.6%	36.4%
	2016	59.4%	35.3%
	2018	55.9%	37.5%
	2019	**70.2%**	**48.3%***

*Exam pass rates by year. * denotes average of first 2 diets of that year*

Reassuringly the 2019 pass rate for MRCP PACES was quite high at 70% and 48% for UK and other trainees respectively.

MRCPUK state that candidates who did not declare their training details are reported as '**other trainees**'. It's presumably fair to assume that this group largely consists of **international medical graduates (IMGs)**, or those who are currently out with a formal training programme.

There are many reasons why 'other trainees' tend to perform less well than their UK counterparts.

Firstly, as this is a British exam, you would expect a larger emphasis on clinical conditions specific to UK clinical practice. This means alcoholic liver disease rather than malaria in the West of Scotland! Having said that, Part 1 still contains many 'weird and wonderful' conditions I've still not encountered in real life.

Another reason for the lower pass rate amongst 'other trainees' is that English may not be their native language. Certain words or phrases that UK graduates take for granted may not be so familiar for international graduates. After all, it makes sense that if you don't fully appreciate the question, or if you take twice as long to read the stem, you're disadvantaged.

This **language barrier** becomes even more pronounced in the final clinical exam, PACES, where candidates are expected to take detailed clinical histories, explain investigations and results, break bad news, in addition to presenting entire cases to examiners under immense time pressure.

To all the IMGs out there I respect all the hard work you've had to endure to join us in the NHS. PLAB alone must've been a headache but this is on an entirely different level.

When referring to exams in general, scores can either be expressed as **raw** or **scaled scores**.

For example, a raw score of 70/100 can also be expressed as 70%. However if we want to compare the difficulty of this exam compared to its predecessor from last year then the raw score isn't very useful.

Let's imagine that we establish that compared to this year's exam, last year's was less challenging.

We introduce a scale from 0 to 300. If a mark of 72/100 last year is deemed equivalent to 70/100 this year by the experts then we assign the same scaled score (for example 220/300) to both marks. This is essentially what happens in the MRCP UK exams.

Instead of a percentage score, candidates are awarded an overall scaled score that ranges from 0 and 999. The current pass score for **Part I is 540**. For **Part 2 it is 454**.

Interestingly, Part 2 pass rates have been historically higher. This could be a result of the lower pass mark required but could also reflect **survivorship bias** – only the best candidates i.e. those who have passed Part 1 are eligible to sit Part 2 written.

Instead of becoming discouraged from attempting MRCP, I hope you'll use all this data to your advantage.

In conclusion, hopefully I've answered how difficult MRCP is. Remember that no matter how impressive they may be, all the registrars and consultants you work with were once in your shoes at some point during their careers.

We were also apprehensive, and uncertainty followed us constantly like a dark cloud above our heads. Numerous consultants told me that failing multiple times prior to success wasn't all that unusual (especially when negative marking existed) and it certainly isn't a reliable indicator of clinical ability.

Part of the battle is having confidence in your own abilities. Compare yourself to yourself from yesterday and not to other people. **Impostor syndrome** is very common amongst medics and I'm quite sure all doctors experience this at some point in their lives.

After all, you've all passed medical school, which is a great achievement in itself.

The difference between attempting and passing

Whilst revising for Part I as a senior house officer, I consulted various registrars and consultants hoping for pieces of wisdom but I was frequently disappointed. Some were only concerned with finishing the ward round. Others chuckled about the number of times they had to re-sit the exam, which didn't help at the time! A few just dismissed the exam as easy - in hindsight they were right but I'm looking at the exam from a completely different angle today, and without other time pressures like ST3 applications.

I was adamant on finding a solution as I think most candidates enter the exam without a plan. After all, if most doctors are clinically sound, why are 50% of candidates still failing? There must be a reason other than lack of knowledge.

One of the most useful conversations I had was with my educational supervisor at the very beginning of core medical training. He advised: "**You must think about MRCP when you eat, sleep and work. Failing is not an option and you shouldn't 'attempt' an exam. You should aim to pass because if you don't, you set yourself back another 3 – 4 months**." He continued: "You end up losing confidence, dignity and you end up lining the pockets of those who charge extortionate exam fees."

The exam fees alone were a deterrent from failing.

My educational supervisor was right and based on his advice I went on to achieve the MRCP diploma in 10 months.

The sooner you attain Part I, the quicker you can attempt Part II written. This will enable you plenty of time to prepare for PACES. If you somehow attain the MRCP diploma early, you can then concentrate on strengthening your applications for ST3 with additional publications, presentations, teaching and quality improvement projects. Moreover, you may wish to use your time effectively by acting up as a medical registrar during CT2.

I'm a big believer in the mantra "work is **not** everything" but achieving landmarks early will give you options. Whether that's geographically, or choice of specialty, these options will open more doors which will in turn give you opportunities that wouldn't have otherwise been possible.

Resources: practice makes perfect

By surviving medical school you've already proven your ability to memorise vast amounts of information. This automatically qualifies you as capable of passing Parts I & II written.

Every student has a slightly different study technique and this can range from rote learning to memory palaces to mind maps. However MRCP is an unusual exam in the sense that if you asked ten doctors for advice regarding resources for Part I, almost all of them will point you in the direction of **practice questions**.

Reading long guidelines can only take you so far and can become terribly dry. If you prefer textbooks then I would recommend *Essential Revision Notes for MRCP by Dr Philip Kalra* and the *Oxford Handbook of Clinical Medicine*.

Like at the start of medical school, many of us may have bought most of the university recommended booklist thinking we need a whole book dedicated on pathology. In reality, we succumb to information overload and analysis paralysis. A better way to study is to use just one reference medical textbook and supplement your reading online or at the library.

If you study like your humble author then I recommend several question banks.

Question banks mentally place you in the clinical situation and can be very useful in the exam and also in clinical practice. It's more realistic and relatable than reading from a textbook and simulates the exam format well. Attempting the question stem followed by a 5-minute light reading session on the answer or the relevant guideline consolidates the information in your mind.

The question bank I recommend above the others is *Passmedicine* as it's cheap and still boasts over 3,000 good quality questions which I couldn't exhaust at the time. The explanations were excellent and followed guidelines to the letter which can be useful for the exam.

For Part I, I'd also recommend *Onexamination*. There are rumours that 5% of the actual exam is based on this question bank! Personally I felt the questions were much more similar to the exam than *Passmedicine*. However the explanations were slightly short at times and I found myself having to drudge through NICE guidelines frequently.

The third popular question bank amongst my peers was *Pastest*. Personally, I would not recommend them as their huge question bank was not neat enough to use. However, I would recommend them for their less well-known video and slide-show lectures.

They contain numerous video or slideshow lectures (by senior registrars and consultants in their fields) on each specialty taking you through their thought processes when tackling various questions. This is a very useful resource to maintain your sanity after doing a few hundred questions...

For Part 2 written I would recommend one book: *Rapid Review of Clinical Medicine for MRCP Part 2 by Dr Sanjay Sharma*. In my opinion, this book is very readable and Dr Sharma takes you through every case as if you were on his consultant ward round. Although the format is not always BOF like in the exam, you should be familiar with the format by now! In this book, hundreds of patient cases are discussed, followed by investigation results and thought-provoking questions.

This mimics the Part 2 Written exam very well and you should familiarise yourself with common investigations including CXR, ECG, and interpretation of a wide collection of blood tests. If you have time to understand rarer investigations such as myocardial perfusion scans or PET scans then I'm impressed! However your return on investment is likely to be very low and chances are you won't use your new found knowledge in clinical practice unless you become a cardiologist or respiratory physician!

This table nicely summarises the main question banks available for the MRCP written exams:

Resource	Cost	No. of questions	App
	MRCP Part 1		
Passmedicine	£30 for 4 months or £40 for 6 months	>3,000	No
Onexamination	Approx. £80 until next exam	3,190	Yes

Pastest	Approx. £80 until next exam	6,700	Yes
MRCP Part 2			
Passmedicine	£30 for 4 months or £40 for 6 months	>2,300	No
Onexamination	Approx. £100 until next exam	1,840	Yes
Pastest	Approx. £80 until next exam	>4,000	Yes

Main question banks for MRCP Parts 1 and 2

The main difference between Part I & Part II written

Although Parts I & II written have a similar format in the sense both exams are BOF, there are some major differences.

If you have prepared adequately you will complete Part I with time to spare. You may even have time to go through every single question again in both papers if you have the stamina.

However in Part II written, even if you have prepared well, finishing on time is an achievement! The question stems are generally twice to three times as long as their counterparts from Part I. There are also numerous investigation results to analyse, all taking up precious minutes.

As a result, I would suggest setting yourself a time limit when tackling questions, especially as your Part II exam approaches. In both exams you're given 1 minute and 48 seconds for each question, or 1 hour for every 34 questions so make sure you time yourself according to this when doing practice questions later on in your preparation.

When doing practice questions, memorising the answers to specific questions is never going to be enough. Firstly, although the MRCP written exams consist of 200 questions apiece, the question bank from which they are taken from are in excess of 30,000 questions. The chances of success using memorisation alone are very slim.

Better is to attempt the full practice question, whilst imagining that you are in the clinical scenario. Attempt the question to the best of your ability and then check your attempt against the best answer. Regardless of whether you answered correctly or not, you should still read the explanations to ensure that your thought process is correct.

If a monkey guessed every question blind-folded it'd still be expected to get 20% of the marks!

Mixed Category Revision

Another important concept to consider is **mixed category revision**. Although there is nothing fundamentally wrong with setting up your revision by specialty when you are doing background reading, it is best to answer practice questions from an unknown category. Let me explain.

If the question stem asks about a breathless patient then this could relate to a cardiovascular, haematological or respiratory condition. If you answer questions based on a specific category e.g. haematology you will have an unfair advantage during practice. In turn this will place you at a significant disadvantage in the actual exam.

Candidates are often worried about their percentage during practice but I'd recommend disregarding this completely. Instead if you're attaining only 40% during practice that means you're increasing your knowledge by a maximum of 150%. This is calculated by the 60% knowledge gap divided by your existing 40% "knowledge". The lower your initial percentage, the more you have to gain from practice questions.

Once you hit 70 – 80% for example, the law of diminishing returns will strike again and you might find that your time will be better spent elsewhere.

Time allocation

One of the main reasons why candidates fail is because they're unable to allocate their time effectively. If you recall the number of marks each specialty is designated, you'll begin to understand that not all specialties are equal. In Part I, clinical sciences is worth 25 marks whilst only 4 marks are allocated to geriatric medicine. This is of utmost importance when deciding how much time you are planning to allocate to each specialty.

To work out how much time you have for each specialty you need to know how many hours you have left to study. Knowing you have 50 days until the exam is not that useful if you're working a busy acute medicine job with 4 upcoming sets of nights and weekends.

Therefore, to get a better idea you must know how many **hours** you have.

If you have 50 days before the next diet and you're planning to revise for an average of 2 hours per day then you should divide the total number of marks in the exam by the total number of hours you have. If you were studying for Part I in this example then 100 hours divided by 200 marks means you can afford to spend 0.5 hours per mark of the exam. Because cardiology is worth 14 marks in the exam this means you can afford 7 hours of your total revision time to cardiology, but only 2 hours to medical ophthalmology, as it's only worth 4 marks.

Most of us would not spend more than 2 hours revising medical ophthalmology anyway, but just 7 hours for a major medical specialty seems ridiculously low. But that is the reality of the matter even when you have "50 days until the exam" in our example. Remember that you are trying to pass an exam so even if you wish to become a respiratory doctor, you should spend no longer than 7 hours on this subject if you have a total of 100 hours to spend. In fact, the astute among you might even spend less time on subjects that you're strong at, and more at your weaknesses...

It doesn't sound like a lot of time but you must be disciplined in the sense you're spending equivalent amounts of time on every aspect of the exam. Otherwise you may find at the very end of your revision you've left some specialties entirely uncovered!

It's important to reiterate that 50 days may sound like a long time for a multiple-choice exam. However even in a 1 in 7 rota you only have 6 free weekends! To put that into perspective, your maximum study time is only a few hours after work and those 12 weekend days. If you factor in long days and night shifts then your time is even less. Do not forget to factor in rest time too as only a lucky few can revise non-stop for 3+ hours.

If you're approaching the exam date with very little time then I recommend spending it on the specialty that you're weakest in and the one that offers most points first. For example if you have clinical sciences and medical ophthalmology uncovered but only have 2 days left, I would recommend spending all your time on clinical sciences.

With random guessing you'd expect 1 mark in ophthalmology and might increase it to 2 or 3 with study and luck of questions. With random guessing you'd expect 5 marks in clinical sciences but could increase it to 15 or 20 with study and luck.

The probability of you encountering questions on clinical science is statistically much higher.

High yield facts & pattern recognition

With stocks and shares a high yield alone does not necessarily qualify the holding as a winner. You may have to consider why the stock or share is yielding such a high dividend - perhaps the business is sinking and is desperate for investors? We also need to consider other aspects such as dividend cover etc.

Thankfully exams are much simpler!

Memorising so-called high yield facts will definitely increase your return on investment. Taking cardiology as an example: a common scenario in the exam is that of the prolonged QTc interval on the ECG. If you spend 10 minutes memorising the main causes such as low electrolytes, various fancy drugs and the genetic conditions your ROI is likely to be very good. Contrast that with attempting to memorise all the different hepatitis C genotypes and their treatment and we know how inefficient the latter approach may be.

It is well known that cramming and superficial learning in this way is not useful in the long term but you will be surprised how much more clinical knowledge you gain and retain by revising this way.

Passmedicine has a good application called the *Knowledge Tutor* which fires a quick series of short high yield questions at you. You can easily answer 100 of them in less than an hour if you don't read the explanations - this is assuming you are looking to quickly test your knowledge as you're approaching the end of your studying.

Another interesting aspect of the exam is pattern recognition. Just as you develop a more "natural" ability to read ECGs the more experience you have the same applies for this exam.

For a simple example in the case of neurology, if the question consists of an overweight female patient who has come to your clinic with a headache then one of your top differentials should automatically be benign intracranial hypertension. If the question supplies extra clues such as papilloedema then you can be even more confident.

One word of warning though - you should still check all the alternative answers and strongly consider the possibility of other diagnoses such as venous sinus thrombosis or intracerebral haemorrhage prior to answering the question.

A good general rule to remember is that in Parts I & II, every piece of information is there for a reason. So if the same lady came to A&E following a head injury then it is probably not BIH!

Variety

Candidates often underestimate the number of hours they need to study to pass Parts I & II. This is probably the second most common reason for failing after poor time allocation.

Although everyone's threshold for concentration varies it is safe to assume that you will need a break eventually. Some people will need more breaks than you and others will need fewer.

Part I is especially challenging for doctors on busy rotas (which is essentially every medical trainee). During this journey you should never be too hard on yourself or feel alone – understand that nobody wishes to study after a hospital shift regardless of how keen or motivated they are. Not to mention that leaving the ward on time is the exception rather than the rule. Then you have the weekends, long shifts and nights on a busy rota. In short, everyone has it tough.

So it is fair to say that one of the attributes of the successful MRCP candidate is grit and determination! Embrace the difficulty of studying for postgraduate exams whilst holding a demanding job and remember that anything worth having never comes easy.

This is where I feel the **importance of variety** becomes paramount in the face of all these obstacles. When motivation is lowest at 7pm on Tuesday night and you find yourself trying to slog through 50 practice questions and their dry explanations. Instead, here is what I suggest.

If you can afford it I would recommend signing up to all three practice question sites. Say you decide to allocate 2 hours of study time every night after a typical 9am - 5pm shift. Split this into 3 separate blocks of 40 minutes each. For the first block (when your motivation is probably at its highest) aim to complete 10 practice questions on your weakest subject and read through their explanations.

That's round 1 - take a break.

A significant number of candidates will probably call it a day by now - I don't blame them and have done so many times. But unfortunately that is a way to fail. However you decide to plod on.

For your second block you complete a further 10 practice questions on your second weakest subject and read through their explanations. If your motivation wavers during any of these two blocks and the allure of that XboxOne/PS4 is just too great, then I suggest reading a completely different topic just to reset things a little. Round 2 done so take another break.

By this time it's getting late. You congratulate yourself but realise you still have one more block. The good news is that this is the block that takes the least effort and willpower on your part. Sit back, open up *Pastest* and watch one of the lectures on either of the topics you are least confident in. Try not to fall asleep.

A more financially savvy way to do this is to use YouTube videos.

Studying for 2 hours per day does not sound like much but it quickly adds up if you are consistent. Most candidates are unable to study for even 2 hours per day and this is reflected on the low pass rate. Nobody likes to study but if you can push through that pain barrier and delay gratification then you'll be rewarded.

The concept is very similar when trying to lose weight or achieve anything practically. Very few people have the motivation to run for 2 hours on the treadmill whereas variety in the form of circuit training makes things more interesting and far less mundane.

This concept should also be used during your weekends off. When your motivation is highest during the mornings you should try to get through as many practice questions and reading in your weakest areas as possible. If your willpower weakens during this, switch to different specialties or reading materials. When you are at your absolute lowest then strategically use those video lectures.

Have a coffee or five.

Stay motivated and keep your chin up - remember that this is only temporary!

Logistics

When I passed parts I and II written, I was on CT1 elderly and acute medicine rotations respectively with full rotas. If you find yourself in this predicament, you will still find the time to study after work if you are dedicated enough!

Some of my more fortunate colleagues did not have on calls for a period of 3 months and used this time to focus on their exam preparation. Although there hasn't been a formal study, it's safe to assume that those with fewer on-calls were more successful in the exam and also in keeping their sanity!

If you do have a graceful period with no on-calls, ensure you use the time to study during this. Once the time is lost you can never have it back.

Another logistical issue to consider is whether you wish to use your annual leave strategically. Some trusts will offer you several days of study leave before the exam for travel and last-minute preparation. I never thought of this at the time, but you can increase your advantage even further by setting 1 or 2 weeks of your annual leave to coincide with the lead up to the exam for maximum gravitas.

This will require discipline and organisation skills on your part but is well worth the consideration. Remember to book study and annual leave early as many of your colleagues may be looking to do the same.

Day of your exam

You will probably have a different pre-exam ritual but my rule was always to stop studying two days prior to the exam. You will find a lot of candidates opening their books in the waiting hall prior to the exam but I was never convinced that last minute cramming helped.

If you adopt the more relaxed approach then remember to keep yourself occupied! There is nothing worse than trying to relax but ending up ruminating (or worse, having nightmares) about the upcoming crime scene. Instead, forget about the exam - easier said than done of course - take a walk, go to the cinema or spend time with your loved ones.

On the day, wake up early and give yourself plenty of time to find the venue.

Settle down. If your exam hall is far away or takes more than 30 minutes to reach then I suggest staying at a fancy hotel the night before. You should do anything that makes your experience easier. Money can always be earned so don't place yourself at a disadvantage by traveling in rush hour for 90 minutes just to save £100 on a hotel.

6 hours is a very long time to keep concentration for and that is one of the reasons why I prefer not to do last minute cramming in the waiting hall. Silly errors as a result of exhaustion would offset the odd mark you would gain from last minute revision anyway.

Keep well hydrated in the morning and make sure you use the bathroom prior to entering the exam hall. You should avoid coffee (unless you really need it for paper 2) and avoid over-hydrating as you will distract your thought process by going to the bathroom.

During the break in between papers, have a light lunch, preferably with candidates who do not discuss questions. Again many candidates will be doing practice questions and fitting in last minute revision. Unless you have superhuman concentration I recommend you do the opposite.

During the two papers, begin with the questions you are most confident with. Then return to the difficult ones and try to make at least an educated guess. Never leave questions blank because there is no negative marking. With BOF questions it is normally possible to eliminate a couple of wrong answers.

My last tip is to have a plan for if you finish early. Although this is unlikely to happen in part II written, finishing with time to spare is common in part I. I would recommend skim-reading all the questions again and ensuring your answers have all been transcribed correctly. I remember picking up two transcription errors in my part I exam this way.

Failing - What Next?

The current UK trainee pass rate for MRCP Part 1 is an abysmal 57.8% so don't beat yourself up too much if you're finding it difficult. If you include all candidates, the picture is even more grim and our collective pass rate falls to 40.2%. One thing for sure is that failing MRCP Part 1 is quite common unfortunately, and in some cases, people fail multiple times.

If you're a UK medical graduate, the statistics above tell us your chances of passing are slightly better than a coin-flip. But we know statistics can be very misleading. The pass rate can easily be skewed towards the right by some very high achievers that exam diet or conversely left by candidates who are only attempting MRCP Part 1 as a box-ticking exercise to get sympathy points at the IMT interview.

Regardless of your current circumstances, here's what you should do if you find yourself failing MRCP Part 1.

Firstly, after a 6-hour exam, I appreciate the last thing you want to do is to sit down and reflect on what the hell happened! But stay disciplined, grab yourself a coffee and at least *consider* the specialty or specialties that really let you down, or gave you a feeling of impending doom.

Confirm this when you get your exam result three weeks later as MRCPUK usually send out a specialty breakdown that looks something like this:

Cardiology	59
Clinical Pharmacology & Therapeutics	20
Clinical Sciences	25
Dermatology	20
Endocrinology, Diabetes & Metabolic Medicine	64
Gastroenterology & Hepatology	45
Geriatric Medicine	90
Haematology	50
Infectious Diseases	60
Neurology	45
Oncology	48
Medical Ophthalmology	0
Palliative Medicine & End of Life Care	70
Psychiatry	67
Renal Medicine	70
Respiratory Medicine	46
Rheumatology	40

Example MRCP Part 1 score

At first glance, that score isn't terrible – could it maybe even scrape a pass? Unfortunately it doesn't.

When we examine the score a little more closely, we realise that the 90% mark we're proud of in geriatrics is only worth about 3.5% of the entire exam! The key is to understand that geriatrics is only worth a maximum of 8 in the 200 marks available in the exam. The other piece of bad news is that our low score in clinical sciences actually cost us almost 10% of the entire exam.

It's natural to read and work on subjects you're already strong at but try and stay disciplined.

The specialty that has the most impact on your score and the one that is your weakest subject should be the target of your focussed study if you find yourself failing MRCP Part 1 or 2. Then focus your efforts on your second weakest and the one that impacts secondarily on your *total score* and so on.

That means that using the above example, I would focus a lot more effort on clinical sciences, haematology, oncology, respiratory, rheumatology and maybe ophthalmology before attempting the exam again.

The next step is to decide when you would reapply. Assuming you've worked reasonably hard for your initial attempt, I would always recommend immediately booking yourself onto the exam at the next earliest opportunity.

Just like a driving test, it would be wise to continue the momentum with driving lessons and book another test immediately. The longer you wait without driving, the less likely you are to pass the next time round.

The only caveat, of course, is if you were completely unprepared on your initial attempt. In that case I would perhaps delay it until the diet after.

Printed in Great Britain
by Amazon

36218971R00026